The Laziest Way to Get Fit and Stay Trim

By Roy Donovan

Copyright

Acknowledgments

Cover design and assistance with digital publishing by K.C. Finn

finn.kimberley4@gmail.com

Preface

Designed for those who are sick of 'slipping back', there are no calorie tables here.

This is for you. No matter what slimming course you are on, it shows you some very revealing facts, and how most people try too hard and get fed up. It is not a large, hard to read book, just an amazing guide packed with details that may hopefully, once and for all, get you onto the right road at last.

So be prepared to get slim and enjoy life!

Table of Contents

Food Intake

We do not need to be fanatical by dieting or measuring calories and so on but, a **prolonged** diet of burgers and chips over a few years would not be conducive to good general health, and also not good for circulation, because of poor **vitamin, mineral and fibre contents**, especially Vitamin E in the case of circulation.

Whereas a reasonable diet where some fruit, vegetables and salads are eaten, preferably daily or several times a week, together with some protein and starches (e.g. cereals or bread). Then this will go a long way to getting into a healthier lifestyle, which may affect **elimination** and also circulation. Trying to eat some granary or wholemeal bread or cereals also gives adequate fibre to assist evacuation and **proper intestinal functioning**.

So when grandma used to ask the children: "Have you had your bowels open?" She was right! By having a daily evacuation of the bowels you should feel much sharper.

The secret is not to try too hard and go completely mad – do not switch all at once to a diet of fruit, vegetables and salads. Your body will most likely not enjoy the shock (neither would mine!). **It is a question of balance**. Some fruit that you like the taste of can be encouraged or increased. The same goes for vegetables. If you don't like a particular vegetable – don't eat it! And if you don't like any vegetables, eat a small amount of them alongside foods that you do like.

You'll still want to eat proteins and carbohydrates such as bread and potatoes of course. And **it may be that you are a vegetarian**, but that doesn't matter, as foods like baked beans are a good source of protein as well as Soya-based meals available from health food stores. Milk and eggs are good protein too, but eggs are best poached or boiled, and only up to 3 a week. Fried may taste good, but they are not good for losing weight.

Obesity

It may be acceptable that one may be up to two stones (or twenty-eight pounds) overweight, however if this weight is increased significantly, especially over a period of years, then this may put a strain upon the body. This may interfere with the circulation and as a consequence may affect the performance of the metabolism of the body.

If you come into this category of person, then my view is **not to go mad** and try to stop everything at once! You will get fed up and **slip back** if you take this approach.

Cut down **gradually** – for example, if you take 3 teaspoonfuls of sugar in your coffee or tea, cut it down to 2 teaspoonfuls until you become accustomed to the new taste (this could take 1 month or so as people's tastes vary). Then when you are used to it, cut it by another teaspoonful, or half teaspoon. At the same time, whilst this is going on, you could also change your ordinary milk, which is most likely full-fat milk, to semi-skimmed. Again, be patient using this method, until you can get onto skimmed milk in your drinks. Now skimmed milk has all the nutrients and minerals, like calcium that ordinary milk has, but it does **not** have Vitamins A and D which are called **Fat Soluble Vitamins**. If need be, you can take a supplement to replace this, an element that we will come to later on.

But while we are on the subject of milk, fat and so on, we will just mention **cheese**. You may be surprised to know that some cheeses have a fat content of 60%, and many have at least 40%. So, if you have been eating a fair amount of cheese up until now, there are two methods for you to consider here. But there is **no need to stop eating cheese**, especially if you like it, as it is a very valuable food.

You could either buy a reduced fat cheese – some cheese fat contents are only 14% (a lot lower than 60% or even 40%). Or, if you really like a particular high-fat brand, then either eat less of it by limiting yourself to once or twice a week instead or five or six times, or (if you want to eat it more often) have much **thinner slices** rather than thick chunks.

The key is to **think about your eating** – if you are a 'chocoholic', for example, cut the frequency down (if you can), but **definitely cut the amount down**. Look for hidden sugar and fat in drinks and packaged or tinned foods. By gradually doing this you will start to lose some excess weight (especially if you start replacing some of these foods with fruits, vegetables and salads).

As for **drinking** – well, we don't want to spoil your social life – but beers and lagers in excess have a lot of calories, so bear this in mind. Try to cut it down somewhat or think of some replacement, for example 'light' beers have reduced calories.

The above may help you to lose weight even if you don't have the time or inclination to do more. However some **exercise** if undoubtedly important if you want to take it one step further. **Walking** takes some beating, not idling along nor jogging, just steady walking for half an hour and at least every other day. Get off your bus 2 stops early, walk the dog more often, whatever it takes. This is paramount to good health.

Other Exercises

Most exercises are generally good for most people, depending upon your **age** and your **condition**. If you are overweight and in bad shape, then do not start a fast or demanding sport. **Consult your doctor** and have your heart and blood pressure checked over before starting a new exercise regime, especially if you are middle-aged plus. If this is the case for you, then walking and **gradually building up the speed and distance** – together with the food intake suggested – may bring about a steady improvement. If you can keep to it, it may stay with you and continue to improve. **Swimming** is also good – regular swimming is a good and gradual strength building exercise.

If you do the above you may find that you do not need or require some of the specific alternative remedies suggested further on in this publication. Also if you do still need the remedies, by using the above fitness methods (generally aiding circulation by walking and/or swimming, watching or controlling your food intake, cutting out smoking etc.) then you may certainly help those remedies to work and tilt your body in the right direction.

Some people are apt to worry greatly, to develop anticipatory anxiety which seems to carry forward to any and every event. So try not to worry, especially as you are now doing something about it. Some people, I have been told, try too hard.

Extra exercises are not absolutely necessary, but can be helpful to get fitter. If you are overweight, middle-aged plus, or just (to be honest) unfit, it's best to only do this now and again to start with, and always consult your doctor if you have any doubts. You could start by doing **wall push-ups**, for example by leaning on any wall and pushing yourself off; do three or four, then the next day but one, four or five, gradually building up. You can extended this to then pushing off say a desk or dressing table, again building gradually, perhaps trying some one-handed push-ups. This is in preparation before moving to full floor push-ups, which can harden up your body and help your strength and image.

Another **helpful stomach hardening exercise** (providing you have consulted your doctor) is to lay on a flat surface, floor or bed. Bend your legs and **just lift your feet off the surface**, only a few inches, and **at the same time lift your head and neck up**. Again if you have lower fitness levels, **start with only one leg**. Breathe in, and upon lifting the leg(s) **hold the position for ten seconds** and start to breathe out, less if you can't breathe out whilst holding the position. Do this two or three times every other day to start with, building up to ten times, then progress to doing this with both legs if you've not already done so. **Do not hold your breath**, as this makes pressure build in your head. Always consult your doctor about any kind of exercise if you have a bad back.

Cellulite and Odema

Cellulite is usually found on the outside of the thighs and is hardly ever found in men. It gives and uneven appearance to the skin, but **here are some tips** on how to reduce it:

1. Massage the area with oils of fennel, juniper, geranium and/or rosemary (available at all good aromatherapy stockists);

2. Increase your intake of water and eat more apples;

3. Cut down on red meat, alcohol and white sugar;

4. Take some Vitamin E to assist circulation, do not exceed the stated dose (as always, if in doubt, consult your doctor);

5. Undertake more walking to stimulate the body, again remembering to consult your doctor again if your fitness levels are low.

Pineapple contains the Bromelin enzyme, which breaks down protein and may assist with cellulite, and also Camellia tea (otherwise known as **Green Tea**) can assist. Green Tea also does not lose many of the useful compounds for general health that ordinary tea does. Green Tea is widely available at health food stores, but establishments like Baldwin's of London (address at the rear of this book) may also have herbal tinctures, fluid extracts and tablet forms.

Odema is excess fluid that is retained in the body tissues, causing swelling, especially in the ankles, under the eyes and around the abdomen. It is best to **consult your doctor if you are on the contraceptive pill**, as this one cause of odema and your doctor may be able to change it for you. There are other causes; however, for example it can be **related to your**

salt intake. You may reduce your salt intake in your food or cooking by buying a **salt replacement** (which may be a type of Potassium); this can satisfy your taste buds without causing any harm.

It is possible to have Osteopathy or Chiropractic manipulation and massage to help with circulation and body metabolism, which helps these conditions as well as your general health, but if you don't have that kind of money to spend you can manage an on-going regime for yourself.

The Value of Walking

If you are in a bad area for walking you could consider investing in a treadmill/walking machine – three quarters of an hour, three times a week does wonders for the body. You should always start gradually – this depends more on your motivation and your diet rather than your age – for example by walking at a normal speed for 5 minutes a day, then in a few days' time in increasing to 10 minutes and so on. You can increase the speed to a brisk walk, but there is no need to run! By the time you increase to between 30 and 45 minutes you should already be feeling generally fitter. If you're finding the routine tedious, remember you can always play music or place your treadmill somewhere where you have a good view to hold your interest.

The benefit of walking only every other day allows the body to rest and muscles to relax and avoid tensing up. The body will also function better in terms of regular evacuation of the bowels through walking, as well as increasing your fruit, vegetables and water intake.

Some Herbalists' Recommendations For Slimming

Nowadays people do not usually start brewing and boiling herbs, although a few still do. You usually buy herbs now in a convenient form, such as a fluid extract or a **tincture**. A tincture is where the herb(s) is preserved in alcohol and you follow the directions to prepare it, for example by pouring hot water that will evaporate the alcohol within a few minutes. You may drink this mixture once or twice a day, depending upon the instructions. Many herbs can now also be bought in tablet form.

Dr Nicholas Culpepper (in his book: *Culpepper's English Physician and Complete Herbal*) recommended **Clivers** to accompany a healthy lifestyle, which is also reputed to be good for the skin. (Some traditional herbalists will recommend Goosegrass instead, which is just another name for Clivers.) They also mention **Seaweed or Kelp tablets** to stimulate the thyroid gland by its iodine content, which is organic. I would suggest, however, that you consult your doctor about such remedies, just in case you have any thyroid abnormalities.

There are many more herbal remedies listed, especially on the internet, however some may not be safe and many have side-effects or bad interactions with prescribed remedies from the doctor, so it is wise not to D.I.Y. a herbal plan for yourself. Always consult a specialist.

Special Conditions for you to Consider

Always consult your doctor about increased physical activity as well as taking Kelp or Seaweed tablets, some organic iodine and some food adjustments.

If you are diabetic then your doctor should already have told you to be careful with starchy foods, carbohydrates and sugar, so when increasing your fruit intake try to avoid sugary fruits like grapes. You may need to produce a list with your doctor of fruits, salads and vegetables that you can have, because in some cases these do have restrictions on them. Also in the general part of this book we have recommended Chromium to stabilise blood sugar levels. Diabetics should especially ask their doctor before taking this.

There are many types of homeopathic remedies, so I have enclosed at the rear of this book the faculty address where you may write or telephone to locate **a doctor who is also trained in homeopathy** in your local area – these are medically trained doctors who are able to give you a homeopathic prescription for slimming.

For British herbalists you should **seek a registered medical herbalist** who is a F.N.I.M.H. (Fellow of National Institute of Medical Herbalists), but this must always be done in conjunction with your doctor if you are on any medication.

Reminders for You – What You Need To Know So Far

You will almost certainly need to cut down, where you can, on **fats, sugar and some carbohydrates**. Don't forget to look carefully for areas of **hidden fat** in foods like cheese and whole milk – get onto skimmed milk in your drink. Also remember that pork is a higher fat meat than chicken and turkey.

Breakfast – If you have cereals for breakfast, have skimmed milk on them instead of whole milk (but remember you can take a vitamin supplement to replace Vitamins A and D that you're losing from the extra fat in whole milk). **Do not mix cereals and toast** – if you do, you are getting the **double starch and carbohydrate** intake. If you are still hungry after your breakfast, eat and apple of something similar.

Snacking – Cut down on mid-morning and mid-afternoon snacks like cakes and biscuits by having fruit instead, for example apples, pears and/or oranges.

Lunchtimes – If you're a fan of sandwiches, watch the cheese! Remember to have salad with it and try fillings like tuna, plus crisps have nearly one-third fat per packet (about 29%) so cut them down.

Evening meals – Have meat with the fat cut off and small amounts of potatoes, rice or pasta with 2 types of vegetables. If you want to lose even more weight, choose fruit here again for dessert with low fat yoghurt, rather than rice pudding or a sticky toffee pudding.

Drinks – Skimmed milk is preferable in coffee or tea, and take plenty of water. Watch your soft drinks – cola has the equivalent of 6 teaspoons of sugar in it, so opt for diet cola instead. Cut down on beer and alcohol in general as it usually has high calories.

Get Walking – It's excellent exercise! For any doubts about exercise, I suggest that you consult a doctor, preferably one who is also a homeopath. As there are many herbs to help with obesity, a Registered Herbalist could help with a prescription.

Stress

Turning to the issues behind problems with diet and exercise, it's obvious that **stress** can play a large part here. Therefore methods to combat stress should be employed to reduce this as much as possible, and for some people this may be no small matter.

Depression and **anxiety** are two more conditions that we have all felt at times, but if we allow these to develop into deeper states and for prolonged periods these can increase the stress on our bodies. This in turn can certainly affect the other parts of the body generally and interfere with physical health.

If you severely troubled by any of the above three, perhaps you could ask your doctor to refer you to a doctor who practices **hypnotherapy**. This may be on the National Health if you cannot afford private fees. Under hypnosis (which is not sleep, but a relaxed state of mind) your mind is said to be more amenable to suggestion. The consultant specialist may be able to bring about significant improvements for you by showing you how to relax your mind and body, and most importantly, how you can keep stress, depression and anxiety from becoming too much to cope with, despite negative conditions.

If you have a small amount of stress, depression and/or anxiety that does not require a doctor's attention – then **simply do your best**. If you can follow this guide and alter some things in your life for the better, then do it. If there are some you cannot, then say to yourself: "What's the point in making myself ill?" If things get you down and you think they're at rock bottom, then there is only one way to go, and that is up.

Anticipatory Anxiety

Anticipatory anxiety is an unpleasant feeling that, more often than not, is much worse than the event that is actually being anticipated. Consider the dental appointment. Some people worry themselves sick – sometimes for weeks ahead of the appointment – others cancel at the last minute, while some just don't turn up. Yet for those that do go, once they are in the chair, it gets better and they wonder why they were so worried in the first place.

Your doctor may suggest **psychotherapy** for this condition. The specialist could talk through your worries and help you to reduce stress and anxiety if this is causing problems in your life. There are alternative methods for stress, anxiety and depression however, it is better if you can **become determined** in your own mind. Make your mind up to take charge of the anxiety and/or negative thoughts, not by suppressing it, but by knowing that it is you who is in control.

There are some people, many people, in fact, who have had all kinds of nasty and severe things happen to them and their loved ones, from bereavement to losing their job and/or business and so on. Bouncing back and making the best of things is unfortunately not so easy for everyone. A **qualified herbalist**, however, could prescribe a few different remedies to help control these kinds of nerves and anxiety issues. Of course, remember to check with a doctor for the possibly of drug interaction.

A doctor who is qualified in homeopathy can be a big help if there are serious problems – these are usually private, however there are a few who work on National Health patients – you may be lucky enough to be referred to one by your doctor if there is one operating in your area. Private doctors, as a rough guide, charge **approximately** £50 for the first session (more in London), the session with involve talking about you and your problems. After the first appointment the doctor may prescribe certain homeopathic tablets for you. These are relatively inexpensive, no more than the cost of a usual prescription, for example £6 to £8 for a small bottle in most cases.

Further Considerations

Homeopathic doctors can treat you for all kinds of conditions we have discussed, including stress, anxiety, depression, high blood pressure, thickened arteries and diabetes.

As there are degrees of **high blood pressure** and also **thickened arteries**, these two conditions often go together – a medical herbalist would quite likely prescribe Hawthorn that works **gradually**, softening the arteries and allowing better circulation, thus allowing the high blood to become more normal. This is **not something you should try to D.I.Y.** yourself, but **what you can do to help yourself** is change some of the red meat in your diet to fish and chicken.

If you were diagnosed as **diabetic** there are alternative treatments for this also. One of the biggest things you can do to help yourself is to understand the basic idea of what's happening in your body – that can help your own doctor or a homeopathic doctor as you will realise how important it is to stick to the diet for diabetics. Very briefly, **the reason for this** is as follows:

Starchy food and carbohydrates in foods such as bread, cake and biscuits have flour in them, as do cereals of all kinds, potatoes and rice. These carbohydrates turn into sugar in everyone, but in diabetes the pancreas does not deal with this quite as it should, hence sugar gets into the bloodstream, causing health risks. This is why diabetic foods have different or alternative sweeteners in them that are not actual sugar; this goes for the chocolate too!

Although there are plenty of addresses where you can obtain herbs and homeopathic tablets for diabetes, I recommend that you **consult a homeopathic doctor first**. The homeopathic dosage for such a complex condition is complicated and a professional will be able to manage it with any other conditions mentioned.

More about Supplements and Doctors

Consider taking a good **Multi-Vitamin/Mineral supplement** that contains Zinc and Vitamin E (consult the listed suppliers at the back of this book if needed). Eat some fruit, salads and vegetables and some wholemeal bread to **help the evacuation of the bowels alongside this**, and to generally feel sharper. Cut down or **stop smoking** if you can, as this **interferes with the circulation**. And remember to cut down on everything **gradually** so you will not slip back into bad habits.

Start more **walking** (after consulting a doctor), especially if you are middle-aged plus of have a weight problem, remembering to do this **gradually** as well. **Do not overdose** on any of the specific remedies listed whilst you're doing this. **Extra does not help** – the remedies would start to cancel each other out. What you are aiming for is a **steady improvement**.

You are allowed to **consult privately** with any of the doctors on the list enclosed, providing that you pay the appropriate fees. If you could not afford their fees (typically around £50), remember to check if they are NHS registered, then you may be able to get a referral from your own doctor, which the NHS then pays for. Most on the list, sadly, are not NHS registered, but this does mean you can consult them without a referral from your own doctor; it's up to you to decide if the fee is worth investing in for you personally.

A Condensation For You – The Top Tips

Providing your doctor has given you the all-clear (if needed), you may select one or more of the following tips to start moving towards a better lifestyle. You may consider starting with drinking 4 cups of water daily. Here are the other tips for your reference:

1. **Do not** change everything suddenly. You will not gain anything by doing this, as you may get fed and slip back, or you may react by having diarrhoea and gastric problems.

2. Gradually introduce a little more fruit, vegetables, and salads into your meals.

3. Gradually cut down on foods like sausages, burgers, chips, pies, cakes, biscuits – cut the frequency down from every day to every other day, and cut the amount down gradually, say from 4 sausages to 3 per meal, and 3 burgers to 2 and so on.

4. Replace foods like sausages/burgers with baked beans or chicken (skin off, or batter off for fish) with a spot of sauce to taste. Salmon or ham (with the fat cut off) are a good idea, and turkey could even replace chicken, as this has even lower cholesterol and lower saturated fat.

5. Gradually replace fried chips with either oven chips, rice or baked potato etc.

6. Replace some of your cakes/biscuits with anything you like from the following: low fat live yoghurt or fromage frais; cottage cheese (get one with something added like chives to give it some taste); apples, pears or even raw carrots.

7. Replace any cream with live yoghurt and/or fromage frais. As for chocolate, try other kinds, for example carob from health food stores, or try to cut down the frequency and amount of your favourite chocolate.

8. Do the walking as stated increasing the time and pace gradually.

9. Do any other exercise you can, e.g. swimming is very good.

With this simple system you are not in a frantic race to lose weight. You can still eat whatever you like, however these guidelines will help you not to go overboard all the time. So if you must, you can still eat the sausages and burgers with a cream cake now and then, but you'll learn not to eat them every day. If you want the best results, practice some of these nine steps every day. This will keep you in charge of your weight loss and your health, rather than being one of these people who has dropped their weight suddenly; it soon comes back on! And more importantly, if people lose weight very fast they often have lasting problems with loose skin, whereas losing weight over time with this gradual method reduces this problem, as the body has more time to adjust to the changes.

Some Ideas For A Menu

On arising, a cup of hot water with cider vinegar.

Breakfast

One banana with low fat live yoghurt OR muesli/Ready Brek.

Mid-Morning

Drink and/or an apple/pear etc.

Lunch

Salad Sandwiches (e.g. lettuce, tomato, beetroot) with any of the following fillings:

Tuna or salmon

Thin slices of cheese (preferably low fat, i.e. 16% fat)

Egg

Chicken

Ham (with fat cut off)

Evening Meal

Carrots and/or broccoli, 2 potatoes/sweet potato, usually with chicken or fish, or occasionally with lamb or beef.

If vegetarian, replace meat with baked beans or Soya protein, with veg as above.

On other days remember to rotate to different vegetables to keep your appetite interested.

Sweet

Fruit, for example melon and/or mango with low fat live yoghurt or fromage frais. On other days rotate to different fruits from the list (overleaf).

List of Foods

Foods to eat more of	Other foods that are necessary	Foods to cut down on frequency and amount
Fruit (in general)	Bread (preferably granary or wholemeal)	Whole or Semi-Skimmed Milk
Vegetables (in general)		Burgers
Salads (in general)		Bacon (cut the fat off to start)
	Eggs (up to 3 times per week)	Sausages
Avocado (high fat, but have		Pies
good fatty acids)	Oats (e.g. porridge or Ready	Cakes
Apricots	Brek), Cornflakes, Special K	Biscuits
Bananas		Sweets
Grapefruits	Milk – preferably Skimmed	Crisps
Melons	(necessary for Vitamins A &	Chips
Mangos	D)	Chocolate
Oranges		Cheese (good protein but high
Pears	Margarine/Low fat spread &	in fat)
Paw Paw	some Butter	Alcohol (high in calories)
Peaches		
	Potatoes	*(The amounts and frequency of*
Beetroot		*these foods is up to you. You do*
Brussel Sprouts	Ryvita / Other cracker	*not have to give them all up,*
Broccoli	products	*just try cutting them down*
Cabbage		*and/or replacing them with*
Celery	Essential Proteins:	*foods from the other columns*
Carrots	Baked Beans	*when you can. Don't put a time*
Onions	Cottage Cheese	*limit on yourself. Enjoy your*
Peas	Low Fat Cheese	*food and take a longer time to*
Broad Beans	Chicken (2-3 times a week)	*reduce amounts. Remember it*
Marrow	Fish (2-3 times a week)	*has probably taken years to put*
Sweet Potatoes	Lamb (once a week if	*on the extra weight, so you'll*
Turnips	desired)	*need months not weeks to*
	Beef (once a week if desired)	*gradually get to the weight and*
Tuna	Tuna (versatile protein, can	*diet balance you want).*
Cottage Cheese	be used in salads and	
Low Fat Cheese	sandwiches too)	
Chicken	Salmon	
Fish	Ham (fat cut off)	

Water – drink plenty	Turkey (can replace chicken)	

Please remember to consult your doctor if you have any allergies or prevailing conditions.

More Books by Roy Donovan

I sincerely hope that this book on getting fit has helped you. If it has, then it would really help me if you would consider leaving a nice review on Amazon and visiting my website at http://www.lifechanginghealth.net and http://roydonovanbooks.com.

You will also find information on other books available through Amazon and the website, such as "*Blood Pressure: Top Ten Tips*" – a practical guide to reducing your blood pressure and getting healthy, and *"Don't Be Afraid of the Dentist Any More"* – which contains techniques and recommendations on overcoming anxiety and fear or dental treatment.

R.D.